The Fertile Garden

Develop Your Family, Develop Your Health

Harmony Royce

DEDICATION

To everyone who, in spite of all the obstacles in life, aspires to inner peace, harmony, and wellbeing. This book provides inspiration, bravery, and resilience for personal growth. I hope these words are a lighthouse for you as you make your way toward a happy and full life.

CONTENTS

ACKNOWLEDGMENTS

The expertise, encouragement, and ideas from many individuals and places came together to produce this book. I want to express my gratitude to everyone who helped make it.

I want to express my gratitude to my friends and family for their unwavering understanding, tolerance, and support throughout this project. Your encouragement has been my inspiration and compass through challenging and creative times.

I am grateful to the readers who have trusted me with their time and attention as they embark on this journey of self-discovery and growth. It is my genuine goal that the wisdom found inside these pages speaks to you and inspires you to design a robust, well-rounded, and satisfying life.

Lastly, I would like to express my gratitude to the entire staff of SmartWave Research Group for their support, direction, and expertise in helping to make this project a success.

With deep gratitude.

CHAPTER 1

THE IMPORTANCE OF FOOD

1.1. The Influence of Nutrition Before Conception

The path to conception is significantly influenced by nutrition, which affects the future baby's health as well as fertility. Healthy eating is only one aspect of preconception nutrition; another is preparing the body for the needs of pregnancy. Why it matters is as follows:

1. Aiding with Fertility: Reproductive health depends on a few key nutrients. For example, folic acid is essential for cell proliferation and DNA synthesis, both of which are required for the formation of a healthy embryo. The omega-3 fatty acids in fish oils boost the health of sperm and the quality of eggs.

2. Hormone Balancing: Hormone regulation, which is essential for ovulation and sperm production, can be

aided by a balanced diet. Hormonal equilibrium is crucially maintained by minerals like zinc and selenium as well as vitamins like B6 and E.

3. Improving Sperm and Egg Quality: Fruits and vegetables that are high in antioxidants shield sperm and eggs from oxidative stress, which can harm DNA and reduce fertility. In this context, antioxidants such as beta-carotene, vitamins C and E, and others are essential.

4. Reducing Inflammation: Persistent inflammation can interfere with implantation and ovulation. Eating foods high in omega-3 fatty acids, nuts, seeds, and leafy greens can help lower this risk.

5. Preconception diet is important because it helps people establish the best conditions for conception and promote the healthy growth of a baby from the beginning.

1.2. Maximizing The Building Blocks in Your Body

The nutrients you eat have a major impact on the cells, tissues, and organs that make up your body.

Here's how to make the most of these foundational elements for a safe pregnancy:

Macronutrients:

These consist of carbs, lipids, and proteins. Each plays a distinct role:

- Semints: Proteins are necessary for the development of the baby's tissues and organs and are also necessary for cell growth and repair. Lean meats, eggs, dairy products, legumes, and nuts are good sources.

- Size: The growth of the baby's brain and nervous system depends on healthy lipids. Walnuts, flaxseeds, and seafood all contain omega-3 fatty acids, which are particularly significant.

- Carbohydrates: These give a developing baby the energy they require. Pay attention to complex carbs, which offer essential nutrients and long-lasting energy. Examples of these include whole grains, fruits, and vegetables.

Micronutrients:

These are vitamins and minerals that are equally important but needed in lesser amounts:

- Folic Acid: Promotes the development of the baby's brain and spinal cord and prevents neural tube abnormalities.

- Iron: Required to produce hemoglobin, which supplies oxygen to the developing fetus.

- Calcium: Vital for the growth of a baby's teeth and bones.

- Vitamin D: Boosts immunological response and improves calcium absorption.

A healthy pregnancy can be achieved by optimizing your body's building blocks through a balanced consumption of these nutrients.

1.3. Diet as Knowledge for a Well-Being Pregnancy

Food provides your body with information that affects hormone levels, gene expression, and general health in addition to serving as fuel. During pregnancy, food communicates with your body in the following ways:

1. Genetics: This field of study looks at how environmental factors, such as nutrition, can impact gene expression. Genes can be turned on or off by specific foods, which can affect your unborn child's health. Folic acid, for instance, can alter how genes important in brain development are expressed.

2. Endocrine Balance: Your hormone levels, which are essential for sustaining a healthy pregnancy, might be impacted by the nutrients you eat. Omega-3 fatty acids, for example, have the ability to modulate prostaglandins, which are hormone-like molecules that affect blood flow, inflammation, and labor induction.

3. The Immune System: An immune system that is stronger in a well-nourished body helps fend off diseases in both mother and child. Zinc and other minerals, as well as vitamins A, C, and E, are important for immunological function.

4. Health of the Gut: Trillions of bacteria make up the

gut microbiome, which is impacted by nutrition and affects immunological response, mood control, and nutritional absorption. A diet high in fiber, prebiotics (found in garlic, onions, and bananas), and probiotics (found in yogurt and fermented foods) can help maintain a healthy digestive system.

By using food as a source of knowledge, you may make decisions that will benefit both your pregnancy and the health of your unborn child.

1.4. Dispelling Myths and Misconceptions About Fertility

There is a lot of false information out there regarding nutrition and fertility. Here, we dispel a few widespread rumors and false beliefs:

Myth 1: Preconception Nutrition Is Only for Women.

- Reality: Both spouses must prioritize nutrition. Diet has an equal impact on male fertility; antioxidants, zinc, and selenium are important for both sperm quality and quantity.

Myth 2: Consuming twice as much food results in a doubled calorie intake.

- Reality: Pregnancy increases nutritional needs, but eating twice as much is not the solution. Rather, prioritize nutrient-dense foods that supply essential vitamins and minerals without being overly caloric.

Myth 3: A nutritious diet can be replaced with supplements.

- Reality: Healthy diets should be supplemented, not substituted, with supplements. Supplements are unable to fully reproduce the diverse mix of nutrients and other beneficial components found in whole foods.

False: All Fat Is Deleted from Fertility.

- Truth: Fertility depends on healthy lipids. For example, the generation of hormones and the quality of eggs depend on omega-3 fatty acids. Replace unhealthy fats from sources like fish, avocados, and almonds with good fats instead of trans fats, which can impair fertility.

Myth 5: Specific Foods Can Ensure Fertility.

- Actual: There is no one food that can ensure conception. Numerous factors, including genetics, lifestyle choices, and general food, affect fertility. Overall reproductive health is supported by a diet rich in different nutrients and well-balanced.

People can make decisions that genuinely promote their fertility and general health by dispelling these beliefs.

Being aware of the significant influence that nutrition has on conception and pregnancy can enable people to choose their food with knowledge. A healthier path to conception and beyond includes preconception nutrition, improving the body's building blocks, seeing food as information, and dispelling myths.

CHAPTER 2

2.1. Using Real Food to Lay the Foundation

Real, whole foods are the cornerstone of any diet designed to increase fertility. These foods are high in vital nutrients and minimally processed, which promotes fertility and general wellness. Why real food important is as follows:

1. Density of nutrients: When it comes to vitamins, minerals, and antioxidants, whole foods have a higher concentration than processed meals. Both general health and reproductive health depend on these nutrients.

2. Decreased Preservatives and Additives: Additives, preservatives, and artificial components included in processed foods can upset hormonal balance and have a deleterious effect on fertility. Whole foods

don't include any of these dangerous ingredients.

3. Improved Blood Sugar Regulation: Whole foods, especially those rich in fiber, aid in blood sugar regulation. The maintenance of hormonal balance, which promotes reproductive health, depends on stable blood sugar.

4. Healthy Fats: Healthy fats are found in whole foods like avocados, nuts, seeds, and fatty seafood. These fats are critical for the generation of hormones and general fertility.

5. Antioxidants: Rich in antioxidants, fruits, vegetables, nuts, and seeds shield sperm and eggs from oxidative stress, a major cause of infertility.

6. Placing genuine food at the center entails emphasizing a wide range of nutrient-dense foods that promote all facets of health and fertility.

2.2. Essential Nutrients for Maximum Well-Being

The main components of a healthy diet are macronutrients, which include proteins, lipids, and carbs. Each contributes in a different way to promoting fertility:

1. Fertility-Related Roles for Proteins: The development and maintenance of all tissues, including reproductive organs, depend on proteins. Additionally, they are essential for the synthesis of hormones and enzymes that control reproductive processes.

2. References: Lean meats, seafood, eggs, dairy products, legumes, nuts, and seeds should all be included. To guarantee a complete spectrum of amino acids, aim for a diversity of protein sources.

Fats

- Participation in Fertility: The synthesis of hormones, cognitive activity, and the integrity of cell membranes all depend on healthy fats. In particular, omega-3 fatty acids are critical for lowering inflammation and promoting the quality of eggs.

- References: Incorporate avocados, almonds, seeds, olive oil, and fatty seafood (such as salmon and sardines). Limit saturated fats from processed meals and stay away from trans fats.

Fats:

- Participation in Fertility: Energy from carbohydrates is required for daily tasks as well as biological processes, such as reproduction. Rich in fiber, complex carbs contribute to steady blood sugar levels.

- References: Give priority to fruits, vegetables, legumes, whole grains (such as quinoa, brown rice, and oats), and veggies. Refined carbs and sugary foods should be avoided as they might lead to hormonal abnormalities and blood sugar increases.

Maintaining the proper balance of these macronutrients guarantees that your body has the building blocks it needs for maximum health and fertility.

2.3. Micronutrients: The Vital Components of Fertility

Although they are needed in smaller quantities, micronutrients like vitamins and minerals are essential for reproductive health. Several essential micronutrients for fertility are listed below:

Role in Fertility:

Folic Acid:

- Cell division and DNA synthesis depend on folic acid. Preventing neural tube abnormalities during the early stages of pregnancy is very crucial.

- Sources: Citrus fruits, legumes, leafy greens, and fortified cereals.

Iron:

- Fertility-Related: Hemoglobin, which transports oxygen to tissues, including reproductive organs, is made possible only by iron. Anemia from an iron deficit might affect fertility.

- Sources: Fish, poultry, lentils, spinach, and red meat. To improve absorption, eat meals high in vitamin C together with plant-based iron sources.

Fertility:
Calcium's Role:

- For healthy bones and the development of a baby's teeth and bones, calcium is essential. It also affects nerve transmission and muscle contraction.
- Sources: Almonds, leafy greens, dairy products, and fortified plant-based milks.

Vitamin D:

- Immune system boost: Vitamin D may help maintain hormonal balance, improve calcium absorption, and boost immunological function.
- Sources: Egg yolks, fortified dairy products, sunlight, and fatty fish.

Zinc:

- Fertility-Related: For ovulation, cell division, and sperm generation, zinc is essential. Additionally, it boosts general health and the immune system.
- Sources: Nuts, beans, seeds, meat, and seafood.

Fat fish, flaxseeds, chia seeds, and walnuts are good sources of omega-3 fatty acids.

Role in Fertility:

Omega-3s lower inflammation, support egg quality, and create a healthy environment for conception.

Making sure you are getting enough of these micronutrients can help you become pregnant and have a healthy baby.

2.4. Fertility Plate Creation: A Balanced and Delectable Dish

Macronutrient balance and a plentiful supply of micronutrients are necessary to create a plate that promotes conception. Here's how to combine everything:

Small Plate Lunch:
- Greek yogurt topped with berries, almonds, and honey drizzled over.
- Nutrient Focus: Antioxidants from berries, protein from yogurt, and good fats from almonds.

Lunch:
- Example Meal: grilled chicken, mixed greens, cherry tomatoes, cucumber, and avocado on top of a quinoa

salad drizzled with lemon juice and olive oil.

- Nutrient Focus: Vegetables provide a range of vitamins and minerals, chicken provides protein, avocado and olive oil provide healthy fats, and quinoa provides complex carbohydrates.

Snack:

- Example Dinner: Hummus-topped carrot sticks.
- Nutrient Focus: Hummus provides healthy fats, protein, and vitamins along with fiber.

Supper:

- Model Dinner: Baked salmon served with sweet potatoes and steamed broccoli.
- Omega-3 fatty acids from salmon, vitamins, fiber, and complex carbs from sweet potatoes are the nutrients that are the focus of this article.

Sweetheart:

- Model Dinner: Dark chocolate with a few assorted fruits.
- Nutrient Focus: Berries and dark chocolate both contain antioxidants.

Surfactant:

- Value: It's important to stay hydrated for both general health and fertility. Try to drink eight glasses of water or more each day. Herbal teas can help you stay hydrated and have other health advantages.

You can prepare delectable meals that enhance your fertility and general health by emphasizing a range of healthy foods and balancing macronutrients and micronutrients.

To sum up, the fertility plate is about intentionally choosing foods that enhance reproductive health rather than just eating properly. A healthy pregnancy can be facilitated by laying a foundation of genuine food, comprehending the functions of macro- and micronutrients, and preparing balanced, nutrient-dense meals. All of these actions can greatly increase fertility.

CHAPTER 3

Putting Your Cycle in Order

3.1. The Hormonal Dance: An Understanding

The intricate interaction of hormones during the menstrual cycle primes the body for pregnancy every month. It is essential to comprehend this "hormonal dance" in order to maximize fertility and general wellness. The menstrual cycle's phases and the hormones involved are broken down as follows:

Days 1–5 of the menstrual cycle:
- Hormonal Activity: Menstruation is the first stage of the cycle, during which the uterine lining sheds. Progesterone and estrogen levels are low.
- Physical Focus: Your body is getting ready for a new cycle by removing the old lining.

Days 1–13 of the Follicular Phase:

- Hormonal Activity: Follicle-stimulating hormone (FSH) induces the production of follicles in the ovaries. A mature one will develop into an egg. The uterine lining thickens as estrogen levels rise.

- Physical Focus: The body is fostering a supportive environment in the uterus and getting an egg ready for ovulation.

Day 14 (Ovulatory Phase):

- Hormonal Activity: A spike in luteinizing hormone (LH) causes the ovary to produce a mature egg. Progesterone begins to rise as estrogen peaks.

- Physical Focus: An egg that is ready for fertilization is released by the body and passes via the fallopian tube.

Days 15–28 of the Luteal Phase:

- Hormonal Activity: The empty follicle develops into the corpus luteum, which secretes progesterone, following ovulation. The uterine lining is stabilized by this hormone, which gets it ready for potential implantation.

- Physical Focus: The body keeps the conditions

conducive to a possible pregnancy. Menstruation results from a reduction in progesterone and estrogen levels caused by infertility.

Nutritional methods to support each stage of the cycle can be more effectively tailored when these stages and their associated hormonal variations are understood.

3.2. Foods to Eat During Your Whole Cycle

Every stage of the menstrual cycle has distinct dietary requirements. Here are some tips for feeding your body during the cycle:

Menstrual Phase:

- Nutritional Focus: Maintain energy levels and replenish lost nutrients.
- Foods You Should Eat: foods high in iron, such as lentils, spinach, and red meat, to replenish iron levels. Foods high in vitamin C, such as bell peppers and citrus fruits, improve the absorption of iron. Warm, calming drinks like herbal teas and hydrating foods like cucumbers and melons can help reduce

cramping.

Follicular Phase:

- Nutritional Focus: Promote egg maturation and increase vigor.

- Foods You Should Eat: Lean proteins, which include fish, poultry, and lentils, aid in the growth of cells. Minerals and vitamins that are vital are found in leafy greens, such as spinach and kale. Nuts and avocados are good sources of fat that aid in the generation of hormones. Brown rice and other complex carbs, such as quinoa, offer long-lasting energy.

Ovulatory Phase:

- Nutritional Focus: Promote healthy reproduction overall and improve egg release.

- Foods You Should Eat: Foods high in antioxidants, such as berries, nuts, and seeds, safeguard the egg and support normal cellular activity. Flaxseeds and fatty fish, which are high in omega-3 fatty acids, help to balance hormones and prevent inflammation. Drinking lots of water and eating meals high in hydration support healthy body processes.

Luteal Phase:

- Nutritional Focus: Manage premenstrual symptoms and support implantation during the Luteal Phase.

- Foods You Should Eat: Foods high in magnesium, such as spinach, almonds, and dark chocolate, can help reduce cramps and mood swings. Potatoes, chickpeas, and bananas are good sources of vitamin B6, which helps with PMS symptoms. Foods high in fiber, such as fruits, vegetables, and whole grains, help with hormone control and digestion.

Optimizing fertility and preserving general health can be achieved by modifying your diet to suit each stage of the cycle.

3.3. Using Nutrition to Treat Common Cycle Irregularities

Many times, cycle irregularities—like irregular periods, heavy bleeding, or intense PMS—can be controlled or improved with targeted dietary approaches.

Here's how to deal with typical cycle problems:

Irregular Periods:

- Nutritional Focus: Help regulate hormones and blood sugar levels.

- Foods to Eat: To balance blood sugar levels, eat whole grains, lean meats, and healthy fats. Steer clear of processed foods and refined sweets as they may lead to hormone abnormalities. Incorporate foods high in omega-3 fatty acids (such as walnuts and salmon) to help regulate hormones and minimize inflammation.

Severe Bleeding:

- Nutritional Emphasis: Restore blood health and replenish lost nutrients.

- Foods You Should Eat: foods high in iron, such as beans, red meat, and fortified cereals, to replenish iron levels. meals high in vitamin C to improve the absorption of iron. foods that are anti-inflammatory, such as fatty salmon, leafy greens, and berries, to lessen inflammation.

Severe PMS:

- Nutritional Focus: Reduce symptoms and promote equilibrium in mood.

- Foods You Should Eat: Foods high in magnesium can help with cramps and elevate mood. B6 to lessen mood fluctuations and bloating. Limit your intake of salt and caffeine, as these might make PMS symptoms worse. Include complex carbohydrates to help keep blood sugar levels consistent.

Through focused nutrition, you can address these problems and enhance both your general health and menstrual health.

3.4. Recipes to Increase Fertility on Every Cycle Day

Fertility-boosting recipes can add flavor and enjoyment to your daily meals while supporting your cycle. For every stage of your cycle, try these recipes:

Menstrual Phase:

Iron-Rich Smoothie

- Ingredients: 1 cup almond milk, 1/2 cup Greek

yogurt, 1/2 cup berries, 1 cup spinach, and 1 tablespoon chia seeds.

- Directions: Mix every item until it's smooth. Savor this iron-rich smoothie to increase energy and restore lost minerals.

Follicular Phase:

- Ingredients: Quinoa and Kale Salad 1/2 cup cherry tomatoes, 1/4 cup feta cheese, 1/4 cup walnuts, 1/4 cup olive oil, 1 juiced lemon, 2 cups chopped kale, 1/4 cup cooked quinoa, and salt and pepper to taste.

- Directions: In a big bowl, combine quinoa, kale, walnuts, feta, and tomatoes. Mix the olive oil, lemon juice, salt, and pepper in another bowl. After adding the dressing to the salad, toss to mix. This salad supplies important vitamins and good lipids to help the egg mature.

Phase of Ovulation:

Seared Salmon with Avocado Salsa

- Components: Ingredients: 2 salmon filets, 1 diced avocado, 1/2 cup diced cherry tomatoes, 1/4 cup diced red onion, 1/4 cup chopped cilantro, 1 juiced lime, and salt and pepper to taste.

- Directions: Use salt and pepper to season the salmon filets. Cook under the grill for 4–5 minutes on each side, or until done. Avocado, tomatoes, red onion, cilantro, lime juice, salt, and pepper should all be combined in a bowl. Present the grilled salmon with avocado salsa on top. This dish offers antioxidants and omega-3 fatty acids to improve egg release and reproductive health in general.

Luteal Phase:

Baked Sweet Potato with Spinach and Chickpeas

- Ingredients: 2 sweet potatoes, 1 can (drained and rinsed) of chickpeas, 2 cups spinach, 1 tablespoon olive oil, 1 minced garlic clove, 1/4 teaspoon cumin, salt, and pepper to taste.

- Guidelines: Turn the oven on to 400°F, or 200°C. Once sweet potatoes are fork-pierced, bake them for 45 to 50 minutes, or until they are soft. Heat the olive oil in a pan over medium heat. Add the garlic and cook it until aromatic. Stir in the cumin, spinach, chickpeas, salt, and pepper. Cook until wilted, about 3 minutes. Once the sweet potatoes are sliced open, spoon the chickpea and spinach mixture on top. This meal helps with PMS symptoms management and implantation because it contains magnesium, vitamin B6, and fiber.

Optimizing your cycle with targeted nutrition can greatly improve your general health and fertility. Supporting your reproductive journey requires understanding the hormonal dance, adjusting your nutrition for each phase, correcting anomalies in your cycle, and integrating foods that increase fertility. You may cultivate a balanced, healthful, and fruitful environment for conception and beyond by making conscious food choices.

CHAPTER 4

COOPERATION IN REPRODUCTION

4.1. Using Food to Support Male Fertility

Male fertility is essential to conception, and fertility is a shared adventure. Sperm health is greatly impacted by nutrition, and specific food choices might increase male fertility. Food can assist male fertility in the following ways:

1. Antioxidants: Sperm DNA damage and decreased sperm count can result from oxidative stress. Free radicals are neutralized by antioxidants, shielding sperm from harm.

Sources: Nuts, seeds, dark chocolate, and fruits and vegetables (including berries, oranges, and leafy greens).

2. Zinc: Both testosterone levels and sperm production depend on zinc. It also promotes general

reproductive health and the immunological system.

Sources: Dairy products, meat, seafood, legumes, nuts, and seeds.

3. Folic Acid: Also referred to as vitamin B9, folic acid enhances sperm quality and lowers the possibility of aberrant sperm development.

Sources: Citrus fruits, legumes, leafy greens, and fortified cereals.

4. Omega-3 Fatty Acids: Sperm motility and general health are enhanced by omega-3s. Additionally, they lessen inflammation, which may have an adverse effect on fertility.

Sources: Walnuts, chia seeds, flaxseeds, and fatty fish (such mackerel and salmon).

5. Coenzyme Q10 (CoQ10): CoQ10 improves the general function and motility of sperm. It prevents oxidative damage to sperm cells by acting as an antioxidant.

Sources: Fish, poultry, meat, whole grains.

6. L-Carnitine: This amino acid increases sperm motility and aids in the synthesis of energy.

Sources: Whole grains, dairy, and red meat.

Men can enhance their fertility and help with a successful conception by including these nutrients in their diet.

4.2 Collaboration and Communication for a Healthful Pregnancy

A supportive relationship and a successful pregnancy depend on partners working together and communicating effectively. Here are some tips for developing a solid alliance:

1. Discussion Open: Open communication about conception and pregnancy can ease tension and foster a caring atmosphere. Talk to each other about your aspirations, expectations, and worries.

2. Common Objectives: Establish shared objectives for your reproductive journey, like stress management, frequent exercise, and eating a balanced diet.

Together, you will fortify your relationship and increase your chances of becoming pregnant by working toward these objectives.

3. Social Assistance: Difficulties with fertility can be emotionally draining. Show compassion and understanding to one another. If necessary, think about getting help from a support group or a counselor.

4. Healthy Lifestyle Decisions: Motivate one another to choose healthy lifestyle decisions, like giving up drinking, stopping smoking, and keeping a healthy weight. Both partners' fertility is positively impacted by these decisions.

5. Consistent Visits: strategy on meeting often to talk about your progress, obstacles you've faced, and any changes your fertility strategy needs to make. By doing this, you can be sure that you will support one another and remain in agreement throughout the process.

Couples can improve their relationship and navigate the reproductive journey more skillfully if they prioritize communication and teamwork.

4.3. Cooking Together and Lifestyle Decisions

A healthy environment for conception and the support of fertility are greatly aided by shared meals and lifestyle decisions.

Here's how to incorporate these elements into your day-to-day activities:

1. Cooking in Unity: Together, you can prepare meals to promote teamwork and guarantee that both partners are following a fertility-friendly diet. Try out new recipes and take pleasure in the cooking experience with your partner.

2. Well-Rounded Diet: Prioritize a well-rounded diet full of entire foods, such as fruits, vegetables, whole grains, lean meats, and healthy fats. Steer clear of trans fats, processed foods, and high sugar.

3. Preparing Meals: Arrange your food so that you get plenty of the nutrients that increase fertility. This may lessen tension and facilitate maintaining a balanced diet.

4. Activity Outside: Stress reduction and preserving a healthy weight both depend on regular exercise. Include things that you both love in your routine, like yoga, dance, or hiking.

5. Handling Stress: Engage in stress-relieving activities together, including deep breathing techniques, meditation, or time spent in nature. Stress reduction can enhance general health and promote conception.

6. Surfactant: To stay hydrated, sip lots of water throughout the day. For both reproductive health and general well-being, enough hydration is crucial.

Couples can foster an environment that is conducive to fertility and general well-being by eating meals together and choosing healthy lifestyle options.

4.4. Establishing a Robust Fertility Group

Developing a successful reproductive team requires working with medical specialists and other resources that can be of assistance.

Here's how to put together a group that will help you on your reproductive journey:

1. Medical Professionals: Select an obstetrician-gynecologist (OB-GYN) or fertility expert who is helpful and well-informed. Any fertility problems can be found and treated with the use of routine examinations and consultations.

2. Dietitians: To support reproductive health, a registered dietitian or nutritionist with expertise in fertility can offer individualized dietary recommendations and meal plans.

3. Experts in Mental Health: Think about consulting with a counselor or therapist with expertise in reproductive health and fertility. They can provide coping mechanisms and emotional support for

handling stress and anxiety.

4. Aiding Organizations: To meet people going through similar things, join online communities or fertility support groups. It can be consoling and uplifting to share tales and counsel.

5. Holistic healers and acupuncturists: Alternative treatments for fertility, such acupuncture or herbal therapy, can be helpful for some couples. Make sure the doctor you select has training in and expertise with fertility treatments.

6. Trainers for Fitness: Creating an exercise regimen that promotes both general health and reproductive function can be made easier with the assistance of a fitness trainer who specializes in fertility-focused exercise regimens.

7. Interaction: Continue to communicate openly with your team regarding fertility. Inform them of your accomplishments, difficulties, and any adjustments you make to your lifestyle or health.

Couples can obtain the assistance and tools need to maximize their chances of conception and preserve general health by assembling a competent fertility team.

Making deliberate decisions to improve reproductive health is a collaborative journey for partners in fertility. Couples can increase their odds of conception and establish a supportive atmosphere for a healthy pregnancy by concentrating on male fertility through diet, encouraging open communication and collaboration, sharing meals and healthy lifestyle choices, and assembling a strong fertility team. This all-encompassing strategy improves partner relationships in addition to promoting fertility, making the path to parenting a fulfilling and shared experience.

CHAPTER 5

5.1. Cycle Charting: Fundamentals

Understanding your fertility patterns and figuring out when you are most fertile requires that you chart your menstrual cycle. You can improve your chances of conception and acquire important knowledge about your reproductive health by monitoring a variety of symptoms and indicators during your cycle.

Here is a step-by-step tutorial on the fundamentals of cycle charting:

A Comprehensive Overview of the Menstrual Cycle:

- Stages: There are four phases to the menstrual cycle: luteal, ovulatory, follicular, and menstrual. There are unique hormonal shifts and fertility indicators with each period.

- Duration of Cycle: The first day of monthly bleeding occurs on day 1 of a typical menstrual cycle, which lasts between 21 and 35 days.

Selecting a Charting Method:

- Paper Charts: Traditionally, daily observations are recorded on a printed chart in paper charts. Books on reproduction and internet resources contain this.

- Apps: Because fertility apps offer easy-to-use digital platforms for tracking and analyzing cycle data, many women prefer to use them. Some of the well-known apps are Glow, Fertility Friend, and Clue.

Menstrual Flow:

- Record the beginning and ending dates of your menstrual cycle along with its strength (light, medium, heavy). These are the Important Observations to Track.

- Basal Body Temperature (BBT): Take a reading of your body temperature before waking up each morning. BBT facilitates ovulation detection.

- Cervical Mucus: Changes in cervical mucus can be a sign of fertility, so keep track of them.

- Cervical Position: A few women additionally take

note of their changing cervical position over the course of the menstrual cycle.

- Symptoms:Keep track of additional signs such as mood swings, breast soreness, or pain during ovulation.

You can easily spot patterns and anticipate fertile windows by keeping a thorough record of your menstrual cycle by charting these observations on a regular basis.

5.2. Comprehending Basal Body Temperature (BBT)

Your body's lowest resting temperature, or basal body temperature (BBT), is determined first thing in the morning before engaging in any physical activity. Because BBT charts make ovulation easier to identify, they are an essential part of fertility awareness.

This is a comprehensive guide to comprehending and monitoring BBT:

How to Determine BBT:

- Apply a Basal Thermometer: A basal thermometer gives accurate readings to two decimal places and is more sensitive than a standard thermometer.

- Regular Timing: Take your BBT each morning at the same time, right after waking up, and before you do anything.

- Action: After putting the thermometer under your tongue and holding it there until it beeps, take a temperature reading.

Pre-Ovulation:

- BBT Patterns and Ovulation: BBT stays relatively low during the follicular phase, usually ranging from 97.0°F to 97.7°F (36.1°C to 36.5°C).

- Stimulation: BBT may drop somewhat right before ovulation and then rise sharply, from 0.5°F to 1.0°F (0.3°C to 0.6°C). This surge signifies the completion of ovulation.

- After Ovulation: Elevated BBT levels continue to be present during the luteal phase, suggesting the presence of progesterone, which raises body temperature.

Reading BBT Charts:

- Coverline: After a few days of charting, create a line

on your chart that indicates the temperature difference between pre- and post-ovulation. The horizontal line that post-ovulation temperatures should fall below is called the coverline.

- Confirmation of Ovulation: Usually, three days in a row with temperatures over the coverline indicate ovulation.
- Structure Patterns: You'll discover patterns over a few cycles that will assist you spot any anomalies and forecast when ovulation will occur.

You can maximize your chances of conception and gain a better understanding of your reproductive window by precisely tracking and interpreting your BBT.

5.3. Cervical Mucus Changes and Fertility Signs

Throughout the menstrual cycle, cervical mucus (CM) undergoes variations in quantity and consistency that are indicative of fertility. Your most fertile days can be identified by tracking these changes and keeping track of them.

Here's a detailed examination of cervical mucus and how it

affects fertility:

Cervical Mucus Types:

- Menstrual Phase: Because of menstrual flow, cervical mucus is not visible during the menstrual cycle.
- Dry Phase: There is usually little to no mucus visible during the dry phase that follows menstruation.
- Stick/Thick: Increased estrogen causes cervical mucus to thicken or become sticky. Sperm motility is less facilitated by this kind.
- Delicious: Cervical mucus becomes creamy or lotion-like closer to ovulation, a sign of increased fertility.
- Egg White (EWCM): When cervical mucus is at its most fertile, it is transparent, elastic, and slick like raw egg whites. EWCM facilitates sperm migration and survival by establishing an environment that is favorable to sperm.
- After Ovulation: Rising progesterone levels cause mucus to thicken and become less plentiful after ovulation.

How to Check Cervical Mucus:

- Observation: Wipe the vagina with clean toilet paper before and after urinating, or stick a clean finger inside to check cervical mucus.
- Recording: Fill up your chart or app with the color, consistency, and volume of mucus that you see everyday.

Fertility Signs:

- Fertile Window: The optimal period for conception is indicated by the presence of creamy or egg white cervical mucus.
- Combined Indicators: For a more precise ovulation prediction, integrate BBT tracking with cervical mucus measurements.

Your ability to recognize fertile days and increase your chances of getting pregnant can be considerably improved by being aware of changes in cervical mucus and their significance.

5.4. Completing the Picture: Understanding Your Chart

It's time to analyze your chart after you've monitored BBT, cervical mucus, and other fertility indicators.

Here's how to assemble every component:

Determine the Fertile Window:

- Cervical mucus and BBT: Peak fertility is indicated by a rise in the BBT and the presence of cervical mucus made of egg whites. Usually, the viable window lasts from a few days prior to ovulation to one day following.
- Day of Ovulation: The day before the BBT rise or the first day of the temperature increase is typically when ovulation takes place.

Cycle Phases:

- Menstrual Phase: Record the beginning of your menstrual cycle and the duration in days.
- Follicular Phase: Record changes in cervical mucus as you monitor the days from the end of your menstrual cycle till the BBT rise.
- Ovulatory Phase: Note the days when the BBT surge and egg white cervical mucus are present.
- Luteal Phase: Track the days after ovulation when

your BBT is increased.

Comprehension of Patterns:

- Standard Cycles: Regular cycles have mucus and BBT patterns that are constant, and ovulation happens around the same time every month.
- Anomalous Cycles: Mucus patterns might be irregular and ovulation days can vary in irregular cycles. Recognizing these anomalies can assist in obtaining medical guidance when necessary.

Using Your Chart for Conception:

- Timing Intercourse: Schedule sex during the fertile window, which includes the day before the BBT rise and days with egg white cervical mucus.
- Projecting Future Cycles: Make plans in accordance with projected fruitful windows by utilizing historical cycle data.

Looking for Assistance:

- Talking with a Professional: For additional assessment, speak with a medical professional or reproductive specialist if you observe any unusual patterns, protracted cycles, or other worries.

You can obtain a better understanding of your fertility and make wise decisions to increase your chances of conception by carefully tracking your cycle and analyzing the data.

Cycle charting, which raises fertility awareness, is an effective technique for comprehending and improving reproductive health. You can more precisely determine your fertile window by learning to measure and interpret additional fertility indicators like changes in cervical mucus and basal body temperature. Not only does this increase your chances of getting pregnant, but it also gives you the ability to make decisions about your reproductive health that are well-informed. Fertility awareness is an important activity that can result in a healthier, more knowledgeable approach to reproductive wellness, regardless of your intentions for conception or just your desire to learn more about your body.

CHAPTER 6

Tracking Tools Optimal for Fertility

Using the correct tracking tools can have a big impact on the process of becoming pregnant. You can now easily and more precisely monitor your fertility with the help of a variety of devices and programs made possible by modern technology. This chapter examines the various kinds of fertility-friendly tracking devices that are available, their functions, and how to pick the best ones for your particular need.

6.1. Cycle tracking technology and charting apps

The way women track their menstrual cycles and fertility has changed dramatically with the advent of charting applications and cycle monitoring equipment. With the help of these tools, you can easily track and evaluate important fertility indicators, gaining insightful knowledge about your overall reproductive health.

Well-liked Charting Applications:

- Key: Clue tracks cervical mucus, basal body temperature (BBT), menstrual cycle, and other reproductive indicators with an easy-to-use interface. It provides predictive algorithms that, when used frequently, become increasingly accurate.

- Friend for Fertility: With a focus on fertility charting, this software offers thorough analysis and interpretations of your cervical mucus, ovulation indicators, and BBT. It has a wealth of educational materials to aid in your understanding of your cycle.

- Ovia: Ovia monitors your menstrual cycle and provides individualized health insights, tracking of symptoms, and fertility forecasts. Additionally, it offers a community forum for guidance and support.

- Shine: Glow provides detailed charting of cycles, logging of symptoms, and fertility forecasts. It also offers individualized health advice and a community of support.

Features to Look for:

- Ease of Use: Consistent data recording is made simpler with an interface that is easy to use.

- Customizability: The flexibility to alter your tracking parameters and monitor a range of symptoms.

- Data Analysis: Applications that offer thorough graphs, charts, and analyses of your data.

- Educational Resources: Read articles, get advice, and get help from the community to understand your fertility better.

You may improve your chances of getting pregnant, understand your menstrual cycle better, and predict ovulation more precisely by using cycle monitoring and charting applications.

6.2. Ovulation Prediction Kits and Fertility Monitors

To track your reproductive window more practically, ovulation prediction kits (OPKs) and fertility monitors are available. These devices provide accurate and timely information about your most fertile days by measuring the hormonal changes that signify ovulation.

Fertility monitor types include:

- Electronic Fertility Monitors: These gadgets monitor variations in estrogen and luteinizing hormone (LH) in the urine. The OvaCue Fertility Monitor and Clearblue Fertility Monitor are two well-liked choices.

- Microscopy of saliva: These gadgets identify alterations in saliva brought on by increased estrogen levels. Saliva takes on a noticeable ferning pattern under a microscope at estrogen peak.

- Ovulation Prediction Kits (OPKs) : The spike in luteinizing hormone (LH) that takes place 24-48 hours prior to ovulation is measured by OPKs. Around the anticipated time of ovulation, they are usually used every day.

Categories of Offspring:

- Based on urine: These kits identify LH in urine using test strips or digital readers. Test strips are not as clear as digital readers like the ones made by Clearblue.

- Based on saliva: These assays identify alterations in salivary composition that point to the impending ovulation and increased estrogen levels.

Using Fertility Monitors and OPKs:

- Consistency: To guarantee reliable results, use the devices consistently and according to instructions.

- Timing: Take the test at approximately the same time every day, preferably in the afternoon or evening when the levels of LH are generally greater.

- Recording Results: To follow trends and forecast ovulation, record your results on a physical chart or in your charting app.

Your ability to time sexual activity for the best possibility of conception is improved by the real-time information that fertility monitors and OPKs provide about your viable window.

6.3. Gaining Fertility Insights with Wearable Technology

A new trend in fertility tracking is wearable technology, which offers continuous physiological parameter monitoring and insights into your reproductive health. These are wearable gadgets that can be used day and night to gather data on different indicators linked to fertility.

Well-liked Accessories:

- Ava Bracelet: In order to determine your fertile window, the Ava bracelet measures a number of physiological indicators, such as your skin temperature, respiration rate, and resting pulse rate. It gives daily insights into fertility and is worn overnight.

- Tempdrop: An upper arm-worn wearable basal body temperature (BBT) monitor is called Tempdrop. Compared to ordinary thermometers, it provides more accurate readings by tracking your body temperature throughout the night.

- Oura Ring: The Oura ring is not just a fertility tracker; it also tracks heart rate variability, body temperature, and sleep patterns, giving important information about general health and wellbeing that may have an impact on conception.

The following are some advantages of wearable devices:

- Continuous Monitoring: Wearables collect data continuously, giving you a complete picture of your physiological changes.

- Convenience: These gadgets are perfect for busy lifestyles because they are light-weight and comfortable to wear.

- Rigidity: When compared to manual tracking methods, wearables frequently yield readings that are more precise and reliable.

How to Use Wearables:

- Consistency: Wear the gadget as advised, usually all day or overnight, depending on the type of device.

- Data Integration: To examine and analyze your data, synchronize the device with the appropriate app or software.

- Pattern Recognition: Make use of the wearable insights to spot patterns and forecast fertile windows.

Wearable technology provides a useful, easy-to-use method of monitoring your fertility, along with insightful information that can improve your comprehension of your reproductive health.

6.4. Selecting the Appropriate Instruments for Your Trip

Your lifestyle, personal tastes, and fertility objectives will all influence which fertility tracking devices are best for you. The following elements should be taken into account while selecting the ideal fertility tools:

Personal Preferences:

- User Interface: Select programs and gadgets that have user interfaces that are simple to understand and navigate.
- Data information: Think about the level of information you wish to monitor and your preference for either automated or manual tracking.
- Support: If you value community features, customer support, and instructional materials, look for technologies that provide them.

Convenience and Lifestyle:

- Time Commitment: If you lead a hectic life, choose low-effort solutions like digital monitoring or wearables.

- Integration: Pick tools that work well together so you can gather all of your reproductive information in one location.

- Portability: Take into account how portable the tools are, particularly if you travel regularly.

Fertility Objectives:

- Precision: If you have problems with conception and require accurate ovulation prediction, think about combining several techniques (e.g., a mix of BBT tracking, OPKs, and fertility monitors).

- In-depth Analysis: When looking at your health and fertility holistically, employ devices that track several physiological markers.

- Medical Guidance: Discuss the best methods with your healthcare practitioner depending on your unique fertility requirements and medical problems.

Expense:

- Budget: The cost of fertility tracking equipment varies, ranging from high-end wearables to free applications. Establish your spending limit and look for tools that provide the most return on your investment.

- Registrations: Apps and services may have subscription costs; be mindful of them and take their long-term affordability into account.

You can select the fertility monitoring tools that will most assist your journey towards conception by carefully weighing these criteria. This will provide you the knowledge and self-assurance you need to manage your reproductive health.

The way that individuals and couples approach their reproductive journeys has changed as a result of fertility-friendly tracking technologies. These gadgets provide useful information and convenience, ranging from wearables, ovulation prediction kits, fertility monitors, and charting applications and cycle tracking technology. You may improve your ability to track your cycle, anticipate ovulation, and eventually reach your conception objectives by learning the features and advantages of each type of tool and choosing the ones that fit your lifestyle and reproductive goals. Accept the role that technology will play in your infertility journey and assume clear, confident control over your reproductive health.

CHAPTER 7

IMPROVING THE HEALTH OF EGGS

A vital component of boosting fertility and increasing the likelihood of pregnancy is optimizing egg health. This chapter looks at the variables that affect egg quality, nutritional approaches to maintain healthy eggs, dietary strategies for specific issues including endometriosis and PCOS, and methods to increase your chances of getting pregnant.

7.1. Comprehending Egg Age and Quality

Quality of Egg:

The ability of an egg to develop into a healthy embryo and its genetic normality are referred to as egg quality. A successful fertilization, implantation, and pregnancy depend on high-quality eggs. Among the elements influencing egg quality are:

1. Chromosomal Integrity: Correct chromosomal

numbers in healthy eggs lower the likelihood of genetic anomalies.

2. Mitochondrial Function: For proper division and growth, eggs need a sufficient amount of energy from their mitochondria.

3. Cellular Health: The viability and developmental potential of the egg are influenced by the state of its cellular environment.

Egg Quality and Age:

1. One of the biggest variables affecting egg quality is age. The amount and quality of a woman's eggs decrease with age because to:

2. Decreased Ovarian Reserve: As women age, their ovarian reserve, which is a limited supply of eggs, diminishes.

3. A Greater Number of Chromosomal Aberrations: As one ages, there is an increased chance of chromosomal abnormalities in eggs, which can result in congenital defects and miscarriage.

4. Decreased Mitochondrial Function: Older eggs may have less functional mitochondria, which affects how well they can develop and supply energy.

Evaluation of Egg Quality:

Even while it can be difficult to evaluate egg quality directly, some markers can offer some insight:

1. Levels of Follicle Stimulating Hormone (FSH): Elevated FSH levels on the third day of the menstrual cycle may signify a reduction in ovarian reserve.

2. Anti-Müllerian Hormone (AMH) Levels: Low AMH levels imply fewer eggs in the population.

3. Antral Follicle Count (AFC): An ultrasound can determine the antral follicle count, which is a measure of ovarian reserve.

7.2. Dietary Techniques to Encourage Healthful Eggs

For the health of eggs to be supported, nutrition is essential. A well-balanced diet that is high in vital nutrients can improve the quality of eggs and the results of reproduction. The following are important dietary tactics:

Antioxidants:

Eggs are shielded from oxidative stress, which can harm

their DNA and biological components, by antioxidants. Antioxidants that are essential include:

1. Vitamin C: Contains leafy greens, berries, and citrus fruits.
2. Vitamin E: Found in vegetable oils, nuts, and seeds.
3. Coenzyme Q10: Whole grains, organ meats, and fatty fish all contain this vitamin.
4. Zinc: Found in legumes, seafood, and meat.
5. Selenium: Found in eggs, seafood, and Brazil nuts.

Omega-3 Fatty Acids:

Fatty acids that are high in omega-3 promote the health of cell membranes and lower inflammation. Among the sources are:

- Fatty Fish: Sardines, mackerel, and salmon are examples.
- Chia Seeds: An omega-3-rich plant-based source.
- Flaxseeds: You can add ground flax seeds to baked goods and smoothies.

Folate:

Vitamin B9, or folate, is necessary for the synthesis and repair of DNA.

- Leafy Greens: like Swiss chard, spinach, and kale are good sources.
- Legumes: Contains black beans, chickpeas, and lentils.
- Citrus Fruits: Includes grapefruits and oranges.

Protein:

Consuming enough protein promotes good reproductive health in general. Opt for lean protein sources like:

- Poultry: Chicken and turkey.
- Fish: Especially those high in omega-3s.
- Plant-Based Proteins: Tofu, tempeh, and beans.

Iron:

Iron is vital for ovulatory function and overall fertility. Include iron-rich meals such as:

- Red Meat: Beef and lamb.
- Leafy Greens: Spinach and kale.
- Legumes: Lentils and chickpeas.

Surfactant:

Proper hydration supports overall cellular function. Aim for at least 8 glasses of water every day, and consider hydrating foods like:

- Fruits: Watermelon, cucumbers, and oranges.
- Vegetables: Celery, tomatoes, and bell peppers.

7.3. Addressing Concerns Like PCOS and Endometriosis with Food

Polycystic Ovary Syndrome (PCOS) and endometriosis are frequent disorders that can influence fertility. Dietary strategies can help address these problems and promote egg health.

Polycystic Ovary Syndrome (PCOS):

PCOS is characterized by hormonal abnormalities, insulin resistance, and irregular menstrual periods. Among the dietary approaches for PCOS are:

1. Low Glycemic Index (GI) Foods: Foods that raise blood sugar levels gradually can assist in controlling insulin resistance. Add non-starchy veggies, lentils, and whole grains.

2. Healthy Fats: Walnuts, flaxseeds, and fatty fish are good sources of omega-3 fatty acids, which can lower inflammation.

3. Anti-inflammatory Foods: Turmeric, berries, and leafy greens are foods that reduce inflammation.

4. Lean Proteins: Fish, poultry, and plant-based proteins help to maintain blood sugar homeostasis.

Endometriosis:

Inflammation and pain are brought on by the proliferation of endometrial tissue outside the uterus in endometriosis. Among the dietary strategies for endometriosis are:

1. Anti-inflammatory Diet: Incorporate plenty of fruits, vegetables, whole grains, and healthy fats.

2. Omega-3 Fatty Acids: Chia seeds, flaxseeds, and fatty fish all help to reduce inflammation.

3. Avoiding Estrogenic Foods: Restrict your intake of processed meats and soy, two foods high in estrogen.

4. High-Fiber Foods: Vegetables, lentils, and whole grains can all aid in controlling estrogen levels.

7.4: Increasing the Probability of Conception

You can use a number of tactics to increase your odds of conception in addition to maximizing egg health.

Timing Sexual Activity:

It's important to know your menstrual cycle and when you're fertile. To find the ideal time for sexual activity, use fertility tracking devices like ovulation prediction kits (OPKs), fertility apps, and basal body temperature (BBT) charts.

- Healthy Lifestyle: Leading a healthy lifestyle can have a big influence on your ability to conceive:
- Maintain a Healthy Weight: Ovulation and egg quality might be impacted by being underweight or overweight.
- Regular Exercise: Hormone balance and general health are supported by moderate exercise.
- Stress Management: Excessive stress has a deleterious effect on fertility. Engage in relaxing activities such as yoga, meditation, and deep breathing.
- Steer clear of toxins: Reduce your exposure to chemicals in the environment that can harm eggs, like plastics and pesticides.

Medical Support:

Consulting with a physician or reproductive specialist can result in tailored recommendations and actions.

- Fertility Testing: Measuring hormone levels, ovarian reserve, and other parameters are examples of potential medical support.

- Medications: Such as ovulation-stimulating fertility medications.

- Assisted Reproductive Technologies (ART): Procedures such as intrauterine insemination (IUI) and in vitro fertilization (IVF).

Partner's Health:

Fertility in men is essential to conception. Encourage your significant other to take up wholesome routines like:

- A balanced diet high in vitamins, minerals, and antioxidants.

- Daily Exercise: Enhances sperm quality and general health.

- Avoiding Toxins: Reducing exposure to hazardous materials and environmental toxins.

- Stress Management: Managing stress by practicing relaxation methods and getting enough sleep.

A holistic strategy is needed to optimize egg health, including knowledge about the effects of aging, nutritional measures, treatment of specific disorders such as endometriosis and PCOS, and lifestyle modifications. Enhancing the quality of your eggs and your overall fertility can help you become pregnant more often and give birth to a healthy child. Accept these techniques to improve your reproductive health and clearly and confidently reach your fertility objectives.

CHAPTER 8

NUTRITION AND HEALTH OF SPERM

Improving egg quality is not as vital as optimizing sperm health because fertility is a shared journey. Healthy sperm are essential for a successful pregnancy, and sperm health can be greatly impacted by a variety of dietary and lifestyle choices. We will explore the vital nutrients that robust sperm require, lifestyle choices that impact sperm health, strategies for assisting your spouse in conceiving, and methods for establishing an environment that is favorable to sperm.

8.1. Crucial Elements for Robust Sperm

Nutrition has a big impact on sperm quality, which includes motility, count, and morphology. Eating a diet high in particular nutrients can help sperm function better and raise the likelihood of a healthy pregnancy.

- Antioxidants: Sperm quality can be impacted by oxidative stress, which can damage DNA. Antioxidants are essential in preventing this from happening.

- Vitamin C: Found in leafy greens, berries, and citrus fruits, vitamin C enhances sperm motility and count while shielding sperm DNA from oxidative damage.

- Vitamin E: Found in nuts, seeds, and vegetable oils, vitamin E lowers oxidative stress to improve sperm motility and general health.

- Selenium: This mineral, which can be found in eggs, shellfish, and Brazil nuts, increases sperm motility and guards against DNA oxidation.

- Coenzyme Q10: Found in whole grains, fatty fish, and organ meats, CoQ10 supports mitochondrial activity, which increases sperm motility and density.

Zinc:

- Sperm motility and count are maintained as well as testosterone production, all of which depend on zinc. Zinc-rich foods include:

- Meat: Lamb, hog, and beef.

- Shellfish: Crab and oysters.

- Legumes: Beans, lentils, and chickpeas.

Carotenoids:

Folate, or vitamin B9, is necessary for the production and maintenance of DNA. Aberrant sperm can result from low folate levels. Among the sources are:

- Swiss chard, kale, and spinach are examples of leafy greens.
- Legumes: Black beans, chickpeas, and lentils.
- Oranges and grapefruits are examples of citrus fruits.

Omega-3 Fatty Acids:

Sperm membrane fluidity and general sperm health depend on omega-3 fatty acids. Among the sources are:

High-Fat Fish: Sardines, mackerel, and salmon.

- Chia Seeds: An omega-3-rich plant-based source.
- Flaxseeds: You may add ground flaxseeds to baked products and smoothies.

L-Carnitine:

The synthesis of energy and sperm motility depend on L-Carnitine, which is present in dairy products and red meat.

Denomination:

Sperm motility and general reproductive health are influenced by vitamin D. Among the sources are:

- Sunlight: Direct sunlight exposure.
- Fat Fish: tuna, mackerel, and salmon.
- Fortified Foods: grains and dairy items.

8.2. Lifestyle Elements that Affect the Health of Sperm

Sperm quality and fertility can be greatly impacted by a number of lifestyle factors. Positive adjustments can strengthen sperm quality and increase the likelihood of pregnancy.

Nutritious Food:

Overall reproductive health is supported by a diet high in fruits, vegetables, whole grains, lean proteins, and healthy fats.

Daily Workout:

Moderate exercise balances hormones and promotes general health, both of which can boost sperm quality.

Excessive activity, though, may have the opposite impact.

Control of Weight:

It's vital to keep a healthy weight. Hormone levels and sperm quality can be adversely affected by being underweight or overweight.

Handling Stress:

Prolonged stress can lower sperm quality and disrupt hormone synthesis. Stress management methods include deep breathing exercises, yoga, and meditation.

Away From Toxins:

Sperm harm can result from exposure to environmental pollutants like chemicals, heavy metals, and pesticides. Exposure can be decreased by staying away from these poisons and choosing natural and organic foods and goods.

Alcohol and Smoking:

Smoking and binge drinking have been related to decreased sperm count and quality. Reducing alcohol use and giving up smoking are two major ways to enhance sperm health.

Temperature Exposure:

Sperm production may be adversely affected by excessive heat. Sunning tight-fitting clothing, saunas, and hot baths can all contribute to maintaining an ideal testicular temperature.

Surfactant:

Maintaining proper sperm production and general health requires drinking enough water. Try to have eight glasses of water or more each day.

8.3. Assisting Your Spouse on Their Fertility Path

Supporting your partner is essential because fertility is a shared journey. Here are some strategies to get involved in the process and make it more enjoyable:

Transparent Communication:

It's critical to keep lines of communication open and honest about your aims, sentiments, and worries. It guarantees mutual understanding and contributes to the development of trust.

Common Responsibilities:

Planning and making decisions on fertility should involve both partners actively. This includes going to doctor's appointments, monitoring reproductive indicators, and changing lifestyle habits together.

Social Assistance:

It can be emotionally taxing to be infertile. By providing patience, understanding, and emotional support, you may improve your relationship and reduce stress.

Well-Being Lifestyle Options:

Making healthy lifestyle decisions as a group helps foster a positive atmosphere. This includes maintaining a healthy diet, getting regular exercise, controlling stress, and abstaining from drugs.

Taking Part in Fertility Treatments:

If you or your partner are receiving fertility treatments, be involved and help them through the procedure. This may entail being aware of treatment guidelines, showing up for appointments, and offering emotional support.

8.4: Establishing a Sperm-Friendly Setting

Establishing an atmosphere that promotes ideal sperm health necessitates the following important actions and ideas:

Nutritious Food and Supplements:
Include a well-balanced meal full of vital nutrients, and if necessary, think about taking supplements. To find the right nutrients to improve sperm health, speak with a healthcare professional.

Avoiding Dangerous Materials:
Reduce your exposure to dangerous substances like chemicals, insecticides, and endocrine disruptors. Whenever feasible, choose natural and organic goods.

Relaxed Activity:
Regularly partake in mild physical activity to preserve hormonal equilibrium and general well-being. Steer clear of intense or excessive activity as it may have a detrimental effect on sperm production.

Stress Reduction:

To promote hormonal balance and general well-being, use stress-reduction strategies like yoga, meditation, and mindfulness.

Maintaining Optimal Temperature:

Steer clear of activities like hot baths, saunas, and wearing tight underwear that might expose the testes to excessive heat. Choose clothing that fits loosely, and take pauses from tasks that require extended sitting.

Consistent Health Examinations:

Make time for routine checkups with your doctor to evaluate your general health and treat any potential issues that can impact your fertility. Results can be enhanced by early detection and intervention.

Improving sperm health is essential to the process of becoming fertile. You can greatly increase your chances of successful conception by learning the critical nutrients required for robust sperm, changing your lifestyle for the better, encouraging your spouse, and setting up an environment that is favorable to sperm. With commitment and hope, adopt these techniques, understanding that each move you take will get you one step closer to reaching your reproductive objectives and creating a happy, healthy family.

CHAPTER 9

DETOXIFICATION BEFORE CONCEPTION

Beyond dietary adjustments, optimizing your health and fertility for conception also entails detoxifying and purifying your body. Here, we look at how important it is to cleanse before being pregnant, how to assist your kidneys, liver, and elimination system, how to establish a sustainable detoxification plan, and mild detoxification techniques for maximum health.

9.1. The Value of Preconception Cleaning

Getting the Body Ready:

The goal of preconception detoxification is to get rid of pollutants that have collected from lifestyle, environment, and food choices. You can improve the interior environment for conception and pregnancy by detoxifying the body.

Toxin Build-Up:

Reproductive health, hormone balance, and general health can all be negatively impacted by toxins. They may build up in the bloodstream, organs, and adipose tissues, which may have an impact on fertility and pregnancy outcomes.

Improving Fertility Potential:

By promoting healthy hormone balance, maximizing nutritional absorption, and bolstering reproductive organ function, detoxifying before conception improves your chances of becoming pregnant.

Reducing Risks:

You can lessen the likelihood of pregnancy-related problems and promote the health of both the mother and the unborn child by limiting toxin exposure and promoting detoxification pathways.

9.2. Moderate Detox Methods for Optimal Health

Whole Foods Diet:

Make the switch to a diet high in fruits, vegetables, whole grains, lean proteins, and healthy fats. Steer clear of artificial additives, refined sugars, and processed foods.

Surfactant:

To enhance kidney function and encourage toxin clearance through urine, drink lots of water and herbal teas.

Fiber-Rich Foods:

To promote bowel movements and improve toxin clearance through stools, include fiber-rich foods such as legumes, whole grains, fruits, and vegetables.

Herbs that Support:

Include detoxifying herbs in your diet or make teas from them, such as burdock root, milk thistle, cilantro, and dandelion root.

Caffeine and Alcohol Limitations:

Limit or completely give up alcohol and caffeine as they can interfere with hormone balance and strain the liver.

Steam or Sauna Treatment:

To encourage sweating and the skin's discharge of toxins, use a sauna or steam room. Drink plenty of water both before and after.

9.3. Encouraging Your Kidneys, Liver, and Removal System

Liver Assistance:

Consume foods high in nutrients and antioxidants to support liver function, such as leafy greens, citrus fruits (oranges and lemons), and cruciferous vegetables (broccoli, cauliflower).

Health of the Kidneys:

Eat foods that promote urine output and have natural diuretic qualities, such as berries, watermelon, cucumbers, and parsley, to improve kidney function.

Hydration:

To maintain kidney function and aid in the excretion of toxins through urine, stay adequately hydrated.

Health of the Colon:

Drink lots of water, eat foods high in fiber, and take probiotics (yogurt, kefir) to support healthy colon function and bowel motions.

Elimination Pathways:

Maintain regular bowel movements, drink enough water, and encourage sweating through physical activity or sauna therapy to support the body's general elimination pathways.

9.4. Formulating a Long-Term Detoxification Strategy

Personalized Approach:

Adapt your detoxification regimen to your lifestyle, food preferences, and present state of health. For individualized advice, speak with a nutritionist or healthcare professional.

Gradual Transition:

To avoid potential detox symptoms like headaches or exhaustion, gradually implement detox procedures and give your body time to acclimate.

Long-Term Shifts in Lifestyle:

Include stress management, eating a balanced diet, drinking plenty of water, exercising frequently, and avoiding pollutants in your daily routine.

Review Development:

Throughout the detoxification procedure, keep track of your development and emotional state. Adapt your plan as necessary to your body's reaction and general state of health.

Safety Precautions:

Make sure the detox program is safe and suitable for your current state of health, particularly if you are on medication or have underlying medical concerns.

Detoxification as a means of conception requires a comprehensive strategy to maximize your fertility and overall health. You can create the ideal conditions for conception and pregnancy by realizing the significance of cleansing, putting gentle detox tactics into practice, supporting your kidneys, liver, and elimination system, and developing a long-term strategy. Knowing that your efforts open the door to a better start to parenthood, embrace this journey with awareness and a dedication to taking care of your body.

STRESS MANAGEMENT FOR FERTILITY

Optimising fertility and increasing your chances of conceiving require effective stress management. Reproductive health and hormone balance can be severely impacted by long-term stress. The impact of stress on conception, relaxation methods to encourage a more tranquil conception journey, resilience building and stressful event management tactics, and fostering a nurturing emotional environment are all covered in this chapter.

10.1. The Effect of Prolonged Stress on Fertility

Integral Dysfunction:

Prolonged stress causes the release of stress chemicals like cortisol, which can upset the delicate equilibrium of hormones involved in reproduction, including testosterone, progesterone, and estrogen. Fertility in general, sperm production, and ovulation can all be impacted by this imbalance.

Irregular Menstruation:

Stress can cause menstrual periods to become irregular, which can alter ovulation's time and regularity. Predicting fertile days and maximizing conception time are more difficult when cycles are irregular.

Decreased In Sexual Desire:

An intimate relationship and regular sexual activity are impacted by stress, which frequently lowers libido and sexual interest—factors that are critical for conception.

Effect on the Health of Sperm:

Stress can lower sperm quality and reproductive potential in males by affecting sperm production, motility, and morphology.

A psychological perspective:

Emotional well-being can be further impacted by stress since it can exacerbate anxiety, despair, and feelings of anger or inadequacy associated with fertility issues.

10.2. How to Relax for a Calmer Travel

Mindfulness-Based Relaxation:

To increase present-moment awareness, lower stress levels, and encourage relaxation, practice mindfulness meditation. Concentrate on practicing body awareness and deep breathing.

Stretching and Yoga:

Yoga is a stress-reduction technique that combines physical postures, breathing techniques, and meditation to increase flexibility and decrease muscle tension. Yoga poses that are gentle are especially good for conception.

Maximum Muscle Relaxation (PMR):

PMR is a technique for promoting deep relaxation and releasing stress by tensing and relaxing various muscle groups. It lessens tension both mentally and physically.

Deep Breathing Exercises:

Relax, lower cortisol levels, and soothe the nervous system by practicing deep breathing techniques like diaphragmatic breathing or box breathing.

Oriented Picture and Illustration:

Conjure up images in your mind of serene, tranquil settings or fruitful outcomes pertaining to fertility by using guided imagery or visualization techniques. Both anxiety and a sensation of control can be enhanced by visualization.

Kinesiology and Acupressure:

Acupuncture and acupuncture are examples of traditional Chinese medicine techniques that can assist regulate Qi, or energy flow, and encourage relaxation in order to lessen the effects of stress on infertility.

10.3. Developing Stress-Reduction Strategies and Resilience

Behavioral-cognitive therapy (CBT):

Cognitive behavioral therapy (CBT) aids in recognizing and altering harmful thought patterns and actions that lead to stress. It encourages coping mechanisms and methods for enhancing resilience.

Time Management and Prioritization:

To lessen overwhelm and better handle stress, develop realistic goals, prioritize your tasks, and plan your calendar.

Community Support Systems:

Keep close social ties with family, friends, or support groups that are cognizant of and sympathetic to your reproductive journey. Seek for emotional support and share your experiences.

Healthy Lifestyle Habits:

Getting enough sleep, maintaining a balanced diet, and engaging in regular physical activity all contribute to general wellbeing and stress tolerance. Steer clear of alcohol and coffee in excess.

Mind-Body Practices:

Take part in mind-body-connection-enhancing activities like journaling, art therapy, or nature walks. Both stress reduction and emotional resilience can be improved by these techniques.

10.4. Establishing an Encouragement-Based Emotional Setting

Open Communication:

Talk to your partner about your feelings, worries, and aspirations around getting pregnant. To build your relationship and offer support to each other, keep lines of communication open and honest.

Achieving Reasonable Goals:

Recognize that there can be ups and downs on the path to fertility. Celebrate little accomplishments along the way and have reasonable expectations.

Gradual Confirmations:

To keep a cheerful and upbeat outlook, engage in self-talk and positive affirmations. Concentrate on your fortitude and ability to overcome obstacles.

Seek Professional Support:

Discuss feelings, coping mechanisms, and relationship dynamics surrounding fertility difficulties with a fertility counselor or therapist. Guidance and validation can be obtained from professional support.

Practices of Self-Care:

Make self-care activities that relax and make you happy a priority. Some examples of these activities include reading, taking a bath, engaging in hobbies, and listening to music. Self-care encourages resilience and emotional health.

Optimizing reproductive health and mental well-being during the fertility journey requires effective stress management. You may face the difficulties of infertility with more positivity and ease if you know the effects of long-term stress, learn how to relax, develop resilience, and create a nurturing emotional environment. Since maintaining your mental and emotional well-being increases your chances of reaching your fertility objectives and creating a happy, healthy family, incorporate these techniques into your holistic approach to fertility care.

CHAPTER 11

BUILDING A HEALTHY MICROBIOME

Building and maintaining a healthy microbiome is crucial for optimizing fertility and overall health. This chapter explores the gut-fertility connection, the role of prebiotics, probiotics, and gut health in fertility, nourishing the microbiome with real food, and addressing gut issues that may impact fertility.

11.1. Understanding the Gut-Fertility Connection

Microbiome Basics:

The microbiome refers to the diverse community of microorganisms (bacteria, viruses, fungi) that reside in the digestive tract, particularly in the gut. This ecosystem plays a vital role in digestion, nutrient absorption, immune function, and hormone regulation.

Impact on Fertility:

A balanced and diverse microbiome is essential for maintaining hormonal balance, supporting immune function, and reducing inflammation—all of which are critical for reproductive health and fertility.

Hormone Regulation:

Gut bacteria influence the metabolism and recycling of hormones, including estrogen and testosterone. Imbalances in gut flora can disrupt hormone levels, potentially affecting ovulation and sperm production.

Inflammation and Immune Function:

An unhealthy microbiome can contribute to chronic low-grade inflammation and compromise immune function, which may interfere with conception and pregnancy.

11.2. Prebiotics, Probiotics, and Gut Health for Fertility

Prebiotics:

Prebiotics are non-digestible fibers found in certain foods that nourish beneficial gut bacteria. They promote the growth and activity of probiotics.

- Sources: Chicory root, garlic, onions, asparagus, bananas, and whole grains.

Probiotics:

Probiotics are live beneficial bacteria that support gut health and balance by crowding out harmful bacteria and supporting digestive function.

- Sources: Yogurt, kefir, sauerkraut, kimchi, kombucha, and other fermented foods.

Supplementation:

Consider probiotic supplements containing strains like Lactobacillus and Bifidobacterium to support gut health. Consult with a healthcare provider for personalized recommendations.

Balancing Gut Flora:

Maintain a balanced microbiome by consuming a variety of prebiotic-rich foods and incorporating probiotic sources into your diet regularly.

11.3. Nourishing the Microbiome with Real Food

Fiber-Rich Foods:

Include plenty of fiber-rich foods such as fruits, vegetables, whole grains, and legumes. Fiber supports digestive health and provides fuel for beneficial gut bacteria.

Colorful Plant Foods:

Consume a diverse range of colorful plant foods rich in antioxidants and phytonutrients. These support overall health and contribute to a balanced microbiome.

Healthy Fats:

Incorporate sources of healthy fats like avocados, nuts, seeds, and olive oil. These fats support gut lining integrity and reduce inflammation.

Bone Broth:

Bone broth is rich in collagen and amino acids that support gut lining health and promote the growth of beneficial bacteria.

Avoid Processed Foods:

Minimize consumption of processed foods, refined sugars, and artificial additives, which can disrupt gut flora and contribute to inflammation.

11.4. Addressing Gut Issues that May Impact Fertility

Digestive Symptoms:

Pay attention to digestive symptoms such as bloating, gas, constipation, or diarrhea, which may indicate gut imbalances.

Food Sensitivities:

Identify and address food sensitivities or intolerances that contribute to gut inflammation and disrupt overall health.

Gut Dysbiosis:

Imbalances in gut flora (dysbiosis) may require targeted interventions such as probiotic supplementation, dietary changes, or gut-healing protocols.

Consulting a Healthcare Provider:

If experiencing persistent gut issues or fertility challenges, consult with a healthcare provider or functional medicine practitioner. They can assess gut health, recommend appropriate testing, and develop a personalized treatment plan.

Building a healthy microbiome is integral to optimizing fertility and overall health. By understanding the gut-fertility connection, incorporating prebiotics and probiotics into your diet, nourishing your microbiome with real food, and addressing gut issues that may impact fertility, you can support optimal digestive function, hormone balance, and immune health. Embrace these strategies as part of your holistic approach to fertility care, knowing that a thriving microbiome contributes to your readiness for conception and a healthy pregnancy.

CHAPTER 12

Sleep and Fertility

In addition to being essential for general health, getting enough sleep is important for conception and fertility. The significance of sleep for conception, methods for establishing a routine that promotes sleep, how to deal with sleep disturbances during the preconception phase, and how to develop healthy sleep habits for the entire family are all covered in this chapter.

12.1. The Value of Restorative Sleep in the Conception Process

Control of Hormones:

A healthy balance of hormones, particularly those necessary for ovulation and sperm production, is maintained by getting enough sleep. Hormones involved in reproduction, such as progesterone, estrogen, and testosterone, can be released when sleep is disturbed.

Menstrual Regularity:

By fostering hormonal balance and guaranteeing appropriate ovulation timing, regular and sufficient sleep contributes to regular menstrual cycles.

Healthy Sperm:

Men who get enough sleep have higher levels of testosterone and healthier sperm motility, morphology, and production.

The Immune System:

Immune system function depends on sleep, which guards against inflammation and infections that may affect fertility.

Reduction of Stress:

Getting enough sleep helps people feel less stressed, which improves their general wellbeing and lessens the damaging effects of long-term stress on fertility.

12.2. Establishing a Sleep-Enhancing Schedule

Regular Bedtime:

To maintain your body's internal clock, or circadian rhythm, set a regular wake-up and bedtime, even on weekends.

Environment for Sleep:

Make a cool, calm, and dark sleeping space for yourself. If necessary, use earplugs, white noise machines, or blackout curtains.

Reduce Screen Time:

A minimum of one hour before going to bed, stay away from screens (computers, tablets, and phones). Screen blue light can interfere with the creation of melatonin, which makes it more difficult to fall asleep.

Relaxation strategies:

Before going to bed, use strategies for relaxation like progressive muscle relaxation (PMR), deep breathing, or mild yoga to let your body know it's time to wind down.

Avoid Stimulants:

Avoid consuming large amounts of caffeine and alcohol,

especially in the hours before bed, as they might disrupt your sleep.

nighttime Ritual:

Create a relaxing nighttime routine to tell your body when it's time to go to sleep, such as reading a book, having a warm bath, or turning on relaxing music.

12.3. Handling Sleep Interruptions Before Conception

Identify Sleep Disruptors:

Determine the elements—such as stress, anxiety, surroundings, or underlying sleep disorders—that are causing sleep interruptions.

Stress Management:

To reduce stress and encourage better sleep, use stress-reduction strategies like journaling, meditation, or speaking with a therapist.

Hygiene of Sleep:

By keeping a regular sleep schedule, establishing a calming nighttime ritual, and improving your sleeping environment, you can practice good sleep hygiene.

Expert Assistance:

Should sleep disturbances continue, speak with a medical professional or sleep specialist to address underlying problems and obtain customized advice.

12.4. Forming Sound Sleep Practices for the Entire Family

Regular Bedtimes:

To promote healthy sleep habits, set regular bedtimes and wake-up hours for both adults and children.

Screen Time Limit:

Establish limits on kids' screen usage and promote calming pastimes like storytelling or reading before bed.

Create a Calm Environment:

Make sure bedrooms have all the elements necessary for a good night's sleep, including cozy bedding, a pleasant temperature, and few outside distractions.

Family Bedtime Routine:

To foster relaxation and camaraderie, establish a peaceful nighttime ritual as a family, such as reading aloud or doing relaxation exercises.

Model Leadership:

Set an example of good sleep hygiene for kids by making sleep a priority for yourself and stressing the value of regular schedules.

For the best possible results with fertility, hormone balance, and general wellness, you must get enough sleep. You may support optimal reproductive health and well-being by understanding the significance of sleep for conception, developing a routine that promotes sleep, treating sleep disruptions during the preconception period, and building healthy sleep habits for the entire family. Accept these techniques as a component of your all-encompassing approach to reproductive care, understanding that a good family life and conception depend on getting enough sleep.

CHAPTER 13

FERTILITY AND EXERCISE

Because it improves overall health, hormone balance, and emotional well-being, exercise is essential for fertility. This chapter explores how to use movement for optimal hormonal health, balance exercise intensity, and design a fun and sustainable exercise program. It also covers establishing the ideal exercise balance for fertility.

13.1. Determining Your Ideal Exercise Balance

1. Individual Needs: When selecting an exercise regimen, be aware of your particular physical state, degree of fitness, and any underlying medical conditions.

2. Consultation: To learn about workout suggestions specific to your health and fertility objectives, speak

with a medical professional or fertility specialist.

3. Types of Exercise: Try out several forms of physical activity, such as mind-body exercises like Tai Chi or Qi Gong, strength training like weightlifting or resistance bands, flexibility training like yoga or Pilates, and cardio exercises like swimming or running.

4. Personal Preferences: To get the most out of exercise for fertility, pick things you enjoy doing and can commit to on a regular basis.

13.2. Exercise for Ideal Hormone Balance

Control of Hormones:

Exercise on a regular basis supports the regulation of key hormones for reproductive health, including cortisol, estrogen, progesterone, and testosterone.

Heart Rate:

Enhancing blood circulation through exercise helps the reproductive organs receive oxygen and nutrients, which supports their health.

Reduction of Stress:

Exercise lessens stress and encourages relaxation, which helps to mitigate the harmful effects of ongoing stress on fertility.

Endorphin Release:

During the fertile journey, physical activity triggers the release of endorphins, which improve mood and general well-being.

13.3. Controlling Activity Level to Boost Fertility

Control:

Steer clear of prolonged or intense activity because these extreme forms of physical strain might throw off the hormonal balance and irregular menstruation cycles.

Be Aware of Your Body:

Observe your body's cues and modify your workout regimen as necessary. Take a nap when you're tired or uncomfortable.

Hyperbolic and Cardiovascular Balance:

Include a well-balanced mix of strength training and aerobic activity to support general health without overstressing your body.

Low-Impact Options:

To reduce joint stress and promote long-term exercise sustainability, think about low-impact activities like walking, cycling, swimming, or light yoga.

13.4. Formulating a Fun and Durable Workout Program

Set Achievable Exercise Goals:

Make sure your fitness level, preferences, and schedule all match together. As your fitness level rises, gradually increase the duration or intensity.

Fun and Variety:

Try new things or enroll in inspiring and motivating group programs to keep your workout regimen interesting and fun.

Coherence:

Make consistency a priority in your workout regimen, aiming for multiple sessions a week to keep up the momentum and reap the long-term rewards.

friendly Environment:

Enlist the help of friends, family, or fellow fitness enthusiasts to help you create a friendly environment for exercise.

Psycho-Somatic Link:

Accept mind-body practices that promote relaxation, lower stress levels, and cultivate an optimistic outlook that supports fertility, such as yoga or meditation.

By increasing overall well-being, improving physical health, lowering stress levels, and supporting hormone balance, exercise is a potent tool for maximizing fertility. You may improve your reproductive journey by determining the ideal exercise balance for your needs, leveraging movement for maximum hormonal health, controlling exercise intensity, and designing a fun and sustainable exercise regimen. Accept exercise as a crucial component of your all-encompassing approach to fertility treatment, understanding that mental and physical well-being are factors in both your preparedness for conception and a successful pregnancy.

CHAPTER 14

FERTILITY AND MINDSET

Your emotional health, stress reduction, and general success of your fertility journey are significantly influenced by the mindset you develop during this process. Here, we cover techniques for developing a hopeful and fruitful outlook, controlling expectations and conquering obstacles, engaging in self-compassion exercises and lowering anxiety, and utilizing affirmations and visualization to increase fertility.

14.1. Fostering an Optimistic and Prosperous Attitude

Psycho-Somatic Link:
Recognize the strong link between mental and physical health and fertility. Develop an optimistic outlook on the possibility of conception and have faith in your body's capacity to conceive.

Thinking Positively:

Affirmations and positive ideas regarding conception, parenthood, and fertility should be the main focus. Shift your negative thoughts to positive and productive ones.

Practice Gratitude:

Every day, cultivate an attitude of abundance, acknowledge the benefits in your life, and turn your attention from difficulties related to infertility.

Backup Plan:

Be in the company of people who will encourage you and who understand your path, such as friends, family, or support groups.

14.2. Controlling Expectations and Getting Past Obstacles

Achievable Expectations:

Have reasonable expectations for the process of becoming pregnant. Recognize that conception can take some time, and be ready for any obstacles that may arise.

Interaction:

Talk honestly with your spouse about your hopes, anxieties, and expectations for getting pregnant. Encourage a unified front as you tackle obstacles as a team.

Empowerment and Education:

Learn about reproductive health, fertility, and available treatments. Gain the knowledge you need to stand up for your needs and make wise decisions.

Seeking Support:

To manage emotional difficulties, process grief or frustration, and create coping mechanisms, seek expert assistance from a fertility counselor or therapist.

14.3. Using Self-Compassion Exercises to Lower Anxiety

Self-Compassion:

Treat yourself with kindness during the process of becoming pregnant. Treat yourself with the same consideration and empathy that you would provide to a loved one going through a comparable situation to demonstrate self-compassion.

Methods for Stress Reduction:

To relax the body and mind, use stress-reduction methods like progressive muscle relaxation (PMR), deep breathing exercises, mindfulness, or meditation.

Healthy Lifestyle:

To enhance general wellbeing and stress tolerance, maintain a healthy lifestyle that includes a balanced diet, frequent exercise, and enough sleep.

Reducing Information Overload:

Restrict your exposure to forums or copious amounts of fertility-related information that could make you feel anxious. When seeking advice, pay attention to reputable sources and dependable medical specialists.

14.4. Fertility Success Visualization and Affirmations

Demonstration Methods:

To visualize a happy ending, try using visualization techniques. For example, picture yourself being pregnant or a safe pregnancy and delivery. An optimistic outlook and less anxiety are two benefits of visualization.

Affirmations:

Compose and repeat positive statements about fertility success, such as "I am deserving of a healthy pregnancy," "I am open to receiving the gift of pregnancy," or "I trust in my body's ability to conceive."

Vision Boards:

Make a vision board that embodies your desires and goals for fertility. Incorporate affirmations, sayings, and pictures that encourage and inspire you to conceive.

Regular Exercise:

To strengthen positivity and resilience, incorporate visualization and affirmations into your daily routine, maybe in the quiet moments before bed or during the morning.

Fertility is greatly impacted by one's mindset, which also affects stress levels, general health, and emotional stability throughout the process of becoming pregnant. You can strengthen your resilience, lessen worry, and foster optimism by developing a positive and fertile mentality, controlling expectations, engaging in self-compassion exercises, and using visualization and affirmations for fertility success. Accept these techniques as essential elements of your all-encompassing approach to fertility care, understanding that mental health has a role in both preparing you for conception and promoting your overall wellbeing during the process.

CHAPTER 15

HONORING YOUR EXPERIENCE

Starting a fertility journey can be difficult, but it can also be life-changing. This chapter looks at how to embrace and help yourself during this journey. Some of the strategies covered are setting up a community of support, assembling a toolkit for fertility, practicing appreciation, accepting the journey, and organizing your next steps to a successful pregnancy.

15.1. Fostering a Community of Support

Value to the Community:

Embrace a network of friends, relatives, or online support systems that are sympathetic to your infertility journey.

Sharing Experiences:

Talk to someone you can trust who can support you, give you advice, or just listen to you about your experiences, feelings, and opinions.

Support Groups:

Take into account joining online or local groups designed to assist people dealing with infertility issues. These communities offer camaraderie, common experiences, and priceless emotional support.

Professional Support:

Seek advice from therapists, coaches, or counselors who specialize in helping individuals and couples with reproductive issues.

15.2. Constructing a Toolbox for Fertility

Educational Materials:
assemble trustworthy data and resources on reproductive health, treatment alternatives, and fertility. Throughout your trip, stay informed to make decisions with confidence.

Health Care Providers:
Build a trustworthy relationship with a reproductive endocrinologist or fertility specialist so they can offer you

individualized care, advice, and needs-based treatment alternatives.

Replacement Therapies:

Investigate complementary and alternative therapies that may enhance general health and reproductive health, such as naturopathy, herbal therapy, and acupuncture.

Nutritional Support:

To optimize your diet for fertility, including foods that support hormonal balance and reproductive health. Speak with a trained dietitian or nutritionist.

15.3. Fostering Appreciation and Accepting the Journey

Practice Gratitude:

Recognize your blessings in life and practice thankfulness in spite of your infertility struggles. Pay attention to the opportunity, love, and support that are all around you.

Cognizance:

Adopt mindfulness techniques to maintain your composure and presence of mind as you pursue conception. Stress is decreased, emotional resilience is strengthened, and a positive outlook is promoted by mindfulness.

Notes:

Maintain a fertility notebook to record your ideas, emotions, and encounters. During trying circumstances, journaling can offer perspective, emotional release, and clarity.

Self-Care Rituals:

Give your physical, emotional, and mental well-being—a high priority—by engaging in self-care activities. Massages, baths, yoga, and time spent in nature are a few examples.

15.4. The Subsequent Actions: Proceeding with Your Path to a Healthful Pregnancy

Continued Planning:

Talk about the next steps in your reproductive journey, such as treatment options, timing factors, and continuous fertility monitoring, with your healthcare team.

Lifestyle Modifications:

To maximize fertility, adopt healthy lifestyle practices like consistent exercise, a well-balanced diet, enough sleep, and stress reduction methods.

Spouse Involvement:

To improve your relationship and support system for each other, include your spouse in decisions and conversations about infertility treatments, emotional support, and lifestyle changes.

Survival and Hope:

As you travel, never lose hope or fortitude. Understand that every step you take toward becoming a parent, no matter what the result, is evidence of your fortitude, tenacity, and dedication.

In order to celebrate your reproductive journey, you should take care of yourself, create a network of support, gather resources, practice gratitude, and face the process with hope and fortitude. You empower yourself on this transforming path by assembling a fertility toolkit, cultivating gratitude, setting up a supportive atmosphere, and organizing the next steps towards a safe pregnancy. Accept every turning point and difficulty as a part of your individual path to motherhood, and know that your commitment and tenacity will lead you to realizing your aspirations of starting a family.

ABOUT THE AUTHOR

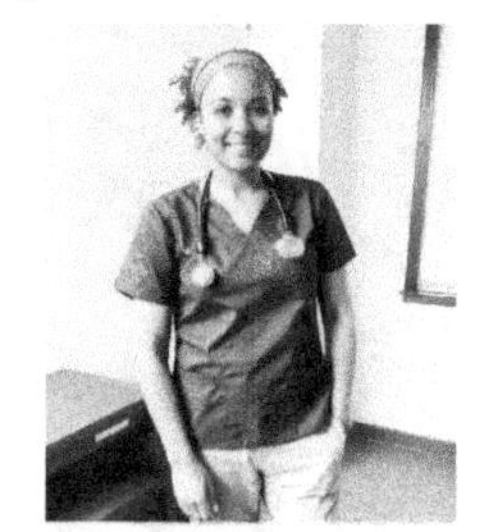 Harmony Royce is a dedicated healthcare worker who has a strong interest in holistic wellness. Harmony's extensive history in various aspects of health and wellness provides her with a wealth of knowledge and expertise that she can utilize in her writing and professional endeavors.

Harmony is a talented author who crafts thought-provoking books that inspire readers to have well-rounded, balanced lives. She writes about a variety of health-related topics, such as diet, exercise, mental health, and mindfulness. Her approachable writing style combines practical guidance with evidence-based research to make complex health concepts approachable and engaging for readers of all ages.

Harmony actively promotes the benefits of holistic health through writing, community workshops, and internet forums. Her mission is to educate and inspire people about the transformative power of self-care and healthy lifestyle choices.